Exploring Diabetes: The Cause and Insulin-Based Treatment

Bob Philz.

Table of Contents

OVERVIEW

There was no disagreement or dispute about which discovery should have won the 1923 Nobel Prize when the scientific committee convened to evaluate the award. The physicians J. and F. G. Banting received the prize. J. R. MacLeod of Toronto for their contributions to the discovery of insulin, and they each promptly gave half of their prize to fellow researchers C. H. Best and J. Collip, B.

Following his return from the war, Dr. Banting was practicing medicine in London, Ontario, and giving a physiology demonstration at Western University's medical school in November 1920. He happened upon a statement in a surgical magazine article that sparked the idea that ultimately resulted in his discovery of insulin, a chemical that gives diabetics a longer and more fulfilling life.

The article he read discussed the pancreas, a gland located near the stomach and upper part of the intestines. It is divided into two parts, one of which secretes an external secretion that is poured into the intestine to aid in food digestion. This secretion contains two other digestive ferments in addition to trypsin. The name "Islands of Langerhans," which comes from the name of the person who discovered them, refers to a distinctive group of cells found in the pancreas that can be distinguished under a microscope from the surrounding tissue.

Diabetes is not a new disease; it has existed for ages.

Ever since the Greek scholar Aretaeus described it in the third century A.D., hundreds of scientists have been working diligently on the issue. In fact, the narrative of insulin's discovery is similar to that of all other significant modern medical breakthroughs. It is the culmination of a great deal of knowledge that scientists from all across the world have slowly but surely contributed. Banting presented his concept to Dr. MacLeod, the University of Toronto's director of physiologic research, as soon as he had it. Seeing the potential in the research, Professor MacLeod gave him a chance to work and paired him with Dr. C. H. Best, a young assistant. The specific issue that needed to be addressed was the extraction of an internal secretion from the pancreas, which the organ had to pump into the bloodstream rather than any other organ or the outside through a dedicated channel.

The substance is secreted by the pancreas; earlier research had suggested that the Islands of Langerhans were the source of its secretion. Trypsin, the external secretion, was known to back up into the pancreas when the tube carrying it was knotted. This occurred because trypsin's digesting effect destroyed the glandular tissue, leaving the organ mostly composed of island tissue.

On a dog, the investigators performed this procedure. It was also recognized that pancreas removal could cause diabetes in an animal; this procedure was carried out on a dog. After enough time had passed for the pancreas in the first animal to break down, the organ was painlessly chloroformed, the pancreas was removed, and an extract was prepared. The diabetic dog received an injection of the extract, which was primarily made of island tissue.

As a result, it was found that the dog's blood and urine contained less sugar after receiving these injections. This and related experiments clearly demonstrated the existence of a substance, absent from the diabetic's body, that was able to meet a deficiency and help the diabetic use sugar appropriately. This substance was most likely found in the pancreas and island tissue.

Medication dosage and animal testing. —It was now required to come up with a way to extract the extract in a pure form that would allow injections into humans without running the risk of poisoning from unneeded and extraneous chemicals. It also became imperative to come up with a way to measure the dosage that was to be administered. How many people who take a medicine dose understand how much research is required to find these factors? Before a drug is tested on a human, it must first be tested on animals. Additionally, to ensure that no unintended side effects arise, it is imperative to thoroughly examine the alterations in the body that occur after the drug is administered.

The Canadian researchers conducted their investigation in an entirely scientific manner. Their experiments demonstrate how well they have considered the controls. There was a normal animal available for comparison with each examined animal. For these essential studies, the investigators used a large number of dogs and rabbits. The medicine was not given to man until every risk factor had been carefully managed. Without the guiding information from the rabbit observations, it appears highly likely that dosages would have been provided and patients would have perished.

Insulin overdose is dangerous.—An excessive insulin dosage can have dramatic effects, including a sharp drop in blood sugar and potentially fatal convulsions. Insulin is a potent medication with definite and precisely quantifiable effects. When someone consumes too much, their blood sugar concentration decreases. He starts to feel self-conscious and frightened when he hits 0.07 percent. He may flush, turn pale, or start to perspire a lot. His speech can become erratic and he might even show signs of mental instability if the blood sugar concentration falls any further. Giving a tiny amount of sugar, such as four to eight ounces of orange juice, can also prevent these things from happening and stop them right away once they do. Experiments carried out correctly also revealed these facts.

Now, the researchers focused on the issue of this illness in humans, and the findings have already been published in newspapers, magazines, and medical journals. They considerably exceed the early expectations of the disease's scientific researchers. Insulin appears to genuinely bring life back when a patient is in the final stage of diabetes, known as a coma, and is losing consciousness. More importantly, it provides comfort and a longer life expectancy for the great majority of diabetics. Because it is well known that the body can process a specific quantity of sugar with the help of a specific amount of insulin, administering it is intimately related to understanding the food that is ingested. To determine the patient's normal ability to digest sugar—which the doctor supplements by administering insulin—the doctor typically requests that the patient come into the hospital before deciding to start the insulin treatment.

Production and distribution: The way that insulin was sold was one of the novel features of its discovery. Although the discoverers were not interested in making an excessive profit from their invention, they were concerned that its mass production and used to be subject to scientific regulation. As a result, plans were developed for it to be produced accurately supervised by the Eli Lilly Company in the United States, Connaught Laboratories in Canada, and, more subsequently, a few additional domestic and international laboratories.

The manufacturing process is a fascinating one. Slightly more than half of this rather small gland is made up of the Islands of Langerhans. This gland is referred to as "sweet bread" in stockyards and packing houses; as these are small, the sweet bread served in restaurants under glass is typically the pancreas of a hog or sheep. At one to one and a half pounds, the beef pancreas is a substantially larger organ.

Collip's technique for extracting insulin from the pancreas entails repeatedly extracting the ground-up organ with alcohol to eliminate extraneous tissue materials. Of course, there is a significant loss of raw materials and compounds utilized in the extraction when this is done on a small scale in a chemical lab.

There were further issues when the substance was applied on a commercial basis. Not only were they successfully conquered, but ongoing advancements have allowed the life-saving treatment to be made available at an affordable cost.

Juvenile diabetes: One of the work's most notable outcomes was the application of the treatment to youngsters with diabetes, or juvenile diabetics. It was once thought that this illness was always fatal. The youngster may now receive satisfactory care, and it appears that the way the medicine is affecting the child could allow for a gradual reduction in dosage to levels that can be given easily and affordably.

Plans were formed for comprehensive clinical research at other institutions where there were men qualified to perform scientific studies on diabetes after the investigators had finished the preparation trials in their hospital. Before being made available to the medical community at large, the drug was subjected to more than 50 institutions for the most comprehensive scientific trial possible. Once these trials were concluded and the collaborating manufacturing concerns had fully developed the machinery for large-scale production of the drug, the drug was made available to the medical community worldwide.

Patients have a responsibility to cooperate with their doctors in order to get the most advantage from this new treatment. It should be known that this cooperation is necessary. He should speak with his doctor about using the medication and eating a healthy diet as soon as a qualified checkup reveals that he is excreting sugar in his urine.

Many times, the patient can live a satisfactory life without insulin if they follow a diet that includes the right quantity of sugar or carbohydrates. In these cases, using insulin is not necessary. In other cases, the insulin dosage might be quite low, but this will be determined after a thorough and thoughtful analysis of each situation.

The general population is now aware that insulin is a preparation that is injected beneath the skin with a needle, a procedure known as hypodermic administration. Because the chemical is digested before it can be absorbed into the circulation, it cannot be taken orally. This does not imply that the patient has to see his doctor for every treatment since numerous skilled professionals who treat this illness have shown that patients can be trained to control their food and take medication as directed.

Acknowledgment of the work: Diabetics rushed to their doctors as soon as word spread about this discovery's availability, asking about the possibility of using it to "treat" their condition. However, the medication is not a "cure" for diabetes in the traditional sense of the word. Diabetes is the absence of specific substances from the body, most likely due to illness, that regulate how sugar is absorbed and used. Insulin cannot replace these tissues or substances, any more than hormone injections can rejuvenate the elderly. It can only momentarily restore the missing substances, but for a diabetic, this can mean the difference between life and death.

Naturally, the world and their peers have bestowed tremendous honors upon Doctors Banting, Best, Collip, and MacLeod. The Canadian government has awarded Dr. Banting $7,500 annually for the rest of his life; the Ontario government has contributed $10,000 annually for a medical research chair, which Dr. Banting is now holding for the first time; and academic societies around the globe have welcomed him with the kind of cheers typically reserved for war heroes.

The garland of the conqueror is undoubtedly worthy of the winner in the battle between science and illness.

FISHBEIN MORRIS.

The etiology of diabetes and its management with insulin

The discovery of a way to obtain insulin in a form appropriate for use in treating diabetes is a reason for true celebration. Insulin is a happy discovery. Remembering this would help you to forgive the exaggerations in the fantastic newspaper and magazine pieces that greeted the finding, which were, in a sense, a public manifestation of such rejoicing. Years have passed while scientists have worked in their labs to try and understand the disease and find a reliable way to control it, all the while the disease continued to claim the lives of more and more young people and the elderly. For example, in New York City, where Dr. Emerson's figures are most trustworthy, there was just one fatality from diabetes out of 2,437 deaths from all causes in 1866. Diabetes was the cause of one fatality out of every fifty-one in 1923. Between 1880 and 1920, the death rate from diabetes in New York City tripled for those up to

45 years of age. It was quintupled for ages forty-five and above. It is likely that there are over a million diabetic patients in the US. Therefore, it seems sense that when word spread that the young Canadians Banting and Best had found insulin, humanity as a whole was ecstatic.

THE DIABETES' NATURE

Diabetes is a metabolic disease. What is insulin and how does it work? Prior to providing a solution, it is necessary to get some understanding of the nature of the chemical problem known as diabetes. This can be achieved by partially reviewing the chemistry and physiology of nutrition.

Most of life's processes include chemicals. Food oxidation and combustion furnish the body with heat. Life ceases and the body cools down in the same way that a gasoline motor cools down when its fuel runs out if the food supply is cut off. In the same way, life will slow down if the mechanisms that convert food into energy are compromised. This is what happens when a person has diabetes; the illness is similar to a motor that fails to ignite when its ignition system is malfunctioning. Similar to gasoline, food too possesses potential energy, which is converted into muscular activity and body heat for life. Diabetes is a disease of metabolism; the systems involved in this conversion are collectively referred to as "metabolism." Although there are other metabolic diseases, none are as prevalent as diabetes.

Carbohydrate, protein, and fat. Humans can only eat plant and animal tissues, and these three substances are used as fuel in these foods: carbohydrates, fats, and proteins. Starches and sugars are considered carbohydrates; oils, lards, and complex substances like brain and egg yolk are considered fats; lean meat and cheese are rich sources of protein. Compared to protein, carbs, and lipids are comparatively simple chemical compounds, fairly stable, and, consequently, easy to analyze scientifically. The word "protein" comes from the fact that they are very malleable. Albumins are a kind of protein. A typical protein with all of the necessary protein properties is egg albumin or egg white. Proteins also construct or restore the body's living tissues in addition to producing energy. Carbs and fats are primarily used as fuels. A diet may be lacking in either fat or carbohydrate and still be adequate. Nonetheless, it needs to supply some protein since the tissues' protoplasmic machinery wears out and needs to be replaced on a regular basis.

Catalysts aid in the disintegration of food. Although the energy found in proteins, fats, and carbohydrates is converted into the life flame through a process of combustion or oxidation, this process involves multiple steps or stages rather than a simple burning or explosion like occurs when fuel is ignited in a gasoline motor. The first of these procedures is carried out in the kitchen during food preparation. There, the proteins coagulate and the carbohydrates soften and partially break down. The subsequent phases of digestion take place when the food moves through the stomach and intestine in turn. They start in the mouth where starches are attacked by ptyalin, a ferment found in salivary juice. Catalysts are another name for ferments. At every stage of digestion and absorption, some catalyst promotes and speeds the process of decomposition in a way comparable to the action of ptyalin on starch, or of yeast in brewing beer. As a result, the meal has chemically broken down into smaller, less complicated pieces than it was when it was first consumed, before traveling more than halfway through the small intestine. The breakdown of starches yields sugars, the most important of which is glucose; the breakdown of lipids yields fatty acids and glycerin; the breakdown of proteins yields relatively simpler molecules known as amino acids.

Sugar in the blood: After digestion, food fragments are absorbed through the intestinal wall and into the blood and lymph, which are the two fluids that flow freely throughout the intestine. If the right chemical techniques are used to identify them, the food fragments can always be found in the blood and lymph. They are highest in the blood in the hours after eating and decrease during fasting. For example, blood drawn early in the morning contains approximately one part per thousand, or 0.1%, of glucose. However, during the digestion of carbohydrates, one and a half parts per thousand, or 0.15 percent, of glucose are detected.

The liver's role: The blood travels straight from the intestine to the liver, where the subsequent phases of metabolism take place. Numerous transformations are carried out in this actual chemical laboratory. Some of these are now known, and here, as in other places later on, there is always a catalyst present to help with each individual chemical shift at every stage of the process. While some catalysts are more broadly active, several are highly specialized and only complete one specific purpose. They have been compared to keys, which allow locks to be turned when they fit into specific locks. It would be difficult for active life, like ours, to exist without these catalysts or accelerators since changes would happen so slowly.

A large portion of blood sugar is extracted by the liver and converted into glycogen, a material that resembles starch. This way, it can be retrieved at a later time when the blood sugar content may be low. The maintenance of a nearly constant blood sugar concentration is one of the liver's primary jobs. It accomplishes this by adding sugar when blood sugar levels are low at night and subtracting sugar when the bloodstream is flooded after meals.

Ammonia separates from the amino acid fragments of proteins in the liver and transforms into urea, a waste product that is subsequently eliminated by the kidneys. Additionally, many protein fragments are used to make sugar, which is then either supplied to the blood or stored as glycogen, which is derived from carbohydrates. Approximately 60% of the protein consumed, measured in dry weight, is subsequently converted to sugar. As a consequence of the liver's action and regular digestive processes, all of the carbohydrates—roughly 58% of the protein and, it is believed, 10% of the fat—end up as sugar.

We need to know the weight of the food as well as how much of it is made up of fat, protein, and carbohydrates if we want to determine how much sugar a particular food will add to our metabolism—that is, its sugar value. The amount that results from adding the weight of the carbohydrates, 58% of the weight of the protein, and

10% of the weight of the fat is the sugar value. For example, a two-ounce (60 grams) slice of bread spread with one-third of an ounce (10 grams). of butter, or 32 grams. six grams of carbohydrates. protein and eleven grams. of fat. This mixture would have a sugar value of 32 + 3.5 + 1.1 = 36.6 grams. 180 grams (6 ounces) of whole milk in a glass. would contain nine grams of milk. 5 grams of carbohydrates. protein and seven grams. of fat, and its sugar value would be around 13 grams, or 9 + 3 plus 0.7.

The blood travels through the liver before entering the heart and being pumped into all of the body's cavities through a network of tubes known as arteries. As a result, fluids that are constantly moving throughout every tissue include sugar and other nutrients in forms that are suitable for consumption energy release in the tissues; no significant chemical changes take place in the blood itself. The tissues take up the food bits from the blood, and within the live protoplasms of each tissue, those crucial alterations take place that make up the most vital functions of life. First, there is the creation of new protoplasmic matter through growth and tissue repair; second, energy is released through more breakdown and ultimate burning or oxidation. Once more, energizers or catalysts are needed at each stage of the change process. Many of these catalysts are just suspected to exist. On the other hand, some of them have been apprehended, and their secrets are now known. Among these is thyroxin, which Kendall demonstrated to be the primary thyroid gland product. Life's speed is set by the thyroid hormone. It regulates the pace of oxygen utilization to such an extent that energy transformation occurs more slowly when the thyroid gland is damaged or absent, as in some cases of goiter.

Now, let's talk about diabetes, a disease that is brought on by a deficiency or absence of the catalyst insulin. It appears that insulin's job is to get sugar ready for use.

Diabetes is a shortage of insulin. Sugar either completely or partially flees the body when it has diabetes. It is essentially "locked up" when the blood flows normally, meaning it cannot be oxidized or undergo any other transformation or stored as glycogen. Its energy is sealed, and you have to turn a lock to release it. Insulin is the key to this lock; without it, the body cannot eliminate sugar from the blood through the usual channels, which causes blood sugar levels to rise and urine to contain sugar.

Diabetes symptoms: Unused sugar accumulates in the blood and excretes in the urine, which is primarily responsible for the symptoms of diabetes. Sugar leaves the body carrying water with it. A patient with diabetes may urinate several quarts every day. This behavior is similar to the process of salt-drying meats or seafood. The body dries out as a result of the water being removed in such large quantities that the tongue may split open and become detached from the roof of the mouth. Furthermore, sugar in the urine causes a significant loss of otherwise accessible dietary energy. A day may see the passing of up to one pound of sugar. As a result, the tissues perish in abundance. As a result, the patient's hunger is heightened; yet, the more food they consume, the more food energy they waste and the worse their symptoms get.

Acid poisoning: This is not the worst case scenario by any means. It so happens that fat, which is easily digested under the right conditions, oxidizes poorly when less than a minimum amount of sugar is used. It is stated that fats burn in the fire of carbs. Certain byproducts of incomplete fat combustion will build up in the body of a perfectly healthy individual if they are fed only fat and very little protein and are not allowed to consume any carbohydrates. These materials are hydroxybutyric acid, acetone, and aceto-acetic acid. While neither acetone nor hydroxybutyric acid are particularly toxic, aceto-acetic acid does behave somewhat like anesthetics like chloroform. When a person has a moderate to severe case of diabetes, burning sugar alone stops the development of acetone bodies, and when a person has severe diabetes, the carbs do not burn.

Diabetic coma: As a result, high levels of aceto-acetic acid may develop in diabetics, potentially causing unconsciousness and anesthesia. This is diabetic coma, which used to be the main reason why young people and children with diabetes died. These coma-related deaths should be avoided with appropriate insulin use.

THE INSULIN STORY

The history of insulin started a generation ago with the discovery made by German researchers Minkowski and von Mehring. This occurred in 1889, and up until then, there was little evidence linking the pancreas to diabetes, and no one knew how to find the tools needed to diagnose the condition. The hand-sized organ known as the pancreas is responsible for secreting digestive juices into the intestine.

Diabetes results from pancreatic removal. Minkowski was researching digestion when it became essential to operate on a dog and remove the organ during some studies. A few days later, it was discovered that this dog's urine was drawing large numbers of flies. After the urine was analyzed, it became immediately clear why there were flies and how the pancreas related to diabetes. There was sugar in the pee. After the pancreas was removed from another animal during surgery, diabetes developed. Then, frogs, pigs, and cats were used in experiments. Every time the pancreas was removed completely, the diabetes was severe; but, when it was removed partially, the diabetes was more chronic and mild.

The Langerhans Islands: In 1869, Paul Langerhans first reported strange cell clusters or islands that are not like the majority of the pancreatic tissue in appearance. By backing up the pancreatic secretions, Scobolew and Schulze (1890) demonstrated that the islands could withstand the damage caused to the rest of the organ when the ducts leading from the pancreas were cut off. It was determined that the islands produced the pancreatic anti-diabetic substance since the animals treated in this way did not get diabetes. The Englishman Shafer proposed the term "insulin" for this substance in 1916.

Previous attempts to produce insulin. Several scientists were working to extract the anti-diabetic component from the pancreas in the interim. A few of these attempts came close to success. Many of these failed because at the time it was unknown that giving insulin orally and allowing it to be broken down by the digestive tract's fluids would render it inactive. Many attempts have been undertakwereto manage diabetes with the use of either freshly harvested pancreas or pancreatic-derived tablets and pellets. Despite the fact that all of these attempts have been ineffective thus far, pharmaceutical companies still market pancreatic pills as treatments for diabetes. More favorable outcomes have been attained by grafting pancreatic segments into dogs whose pancreas had previously been removed to induce diabetes. It is possible to regulate experimental diabetes in animals receiving this treatment, but human benefit from such operations is negligible as grafts from lower animals to humans always diminish and eventually disappear.

Banting's idea: This was the situation when Frederick Banting, who had just returned from the war, started working on the subject in the fall of 1920. He claims that while reading an article about the connection between diabetes and the islands of Langerhans, the idea struck. According to him, it was as follows: "The idea presented itself that since the acinous, but not the islet tissue, degenerates after this operation, advantage might be taken of this fact to prepare an active extract of islet tissue. This is based on the passage in this article that gives a resumé of degenerative changes in the acini (cells connected with the ducts or passageway system) of the pancreas." The secondary theory postulated that trypsinogen, a digestive ferment produced by acinous cells, or its byproducts acted as an antagonist to the gland's internal secretion. Thus, Banting reasoned that the failures of his predecessors in this heavily researched field could be explained by the likelihood that the pancreatic digestive juices would destroy insulin before it could be extracted from the islands. His strategy was to get around this problem by first eliminating the portion of the pancreas that was responsible for producing these juices.

Banting presented his concept to University of Toronto Professor Macleod, who created the first insulin. He was given support and workspace, and he tested the idea in Professor Macleod's lab with the expert guidance of Mr. C. H. Best. The experiment was successful. Dogs with diabetes that had had their pancreas removed could still live because they were given treatment using tissue from degenerating pancreas. Every time this substance was injected under the skin, the amount of sugar in their urine also dropped and the amount of sugar in their blood decreased. The original insulin was this one. Not long after, the next action was taken. The pancreas of animals in the womb, that is, of embryos or fetuses, exhibits island tissue at some point in their development before the tissue responsible for the digestive fluids is fully formed, as Banting and Best knew from the work of their predecessors. Hence, it dawned on them that they could produce insulin from embryo calves, thereby avoiding the damaging effects of the juices. When attempted, this worked well. There was enough insulin to test on a patient. Subsequent advancements made it possible to prepare insulin from mature animals. Insulin was first produced from the pancreas of cattle and pigs that were killed. These preparations were initially toxic due to the presence of protein, making them unfit for usage in patients. Professor J. B. Collip, a chemist at the University of Toronto, successfully surmounted this challenge. With the help of several skilled medical professionals, including Doctors Graham, Campbell, and Fletcher, the novel insulin was administered to a sizable patient population, establishing its proven benefits.

Insulin is now accessible to all.—Thanks to smart arrangements for preserving control over its production made possible by the University of Toronto, insulin is now available in every pharmacy and, thankfully, is always of uniform potency. The most crucial issue is this one of continuous strength. Its indiscriminate use is dangerous, as will become clear later, and the dosage needs to be adjusted to correspond with the amount of sugar that can be obtained via food. Accurate treatment would not be possible unless the strength of different lots of insulin remained constant. Workers in Toronto became aware of this early on, and in order to safeguard the public, it was determined that insulin needed to be trademarked. This would allow the production of insulin to be limited to companies willing to allow an insulin committee in Toronto to oversee their goods. The Indianapolis-based Eli Lilly and Company offered the committee access to their facilities and helped establish large-scale production techniques. The insulin committee has since granted licenses to additional businesses to produce insulin.

The majority of doctors disapprove of their findings being patented. It goes against the profession's code of ethics. However, the patenting of insulin does not go against this code of ethics because, although it was obtained in the names of Doctor Banting and his associates, the patent was given to the University of Toronto outright to be used for the purpose of ensuring that this wonderful discovery would not be used by others to its detriment rather than for any commercial advantage.

Described as follows: Insulin is now sold as a transparent, diluted solution. 50, 100, or 200 units are contained in a tiny vial, depending on the label. The unit's strength is typical. An animal in normalcy will see a clear reduction in blood sugar levels after taking one unit of insulin. The test animal of choice is the rabbit. Depending on the nature of the diet and the existence or absence of problems, an insulin unit will boost tolerance in a diabetic patient, increasing the quantity of sugar that can be used from 0.5 grams to 4 grams. The typical patient consumes ten to thirty units per day on average. Insulin can now be purchased for less than one penny per unit, making it more affordable for all. When we take into account that patients who were helpless invalids reliant on family or charity before receiving insulin are now as robust and fit as their neighbors and are able to return to work, the cost is actually small.

THE DIABETES CAUSE

Diabetes is brought on by pancreatic disease. The pancreas, which is situated in the abdomen next to the stomach and secretes digestive juices into the intestine through a duct or channel, is what Minkowski demonstrated to be the cause of diabetes. As was previously mentioned, the organ also has a secondary purpose, which is to produce insulin. This second product enters the bloodstream after being refined by the Langerhans islets. It is appropriate to consider the Langerhans islands to be a unique organ. But since they are so closely linked to and integrated with the rest of the pancreas, any illness or damage to the organ can have a significant impact on them, lowering their ability to produce insulin and ultimately leading to diabetes. Actually, before diabetes manifests, the pancreas may be largely gone. In dogs, it takes no more than 10 percent of the gland to remain intact in order to stop sugar from being excreted. Compared to dogs, men are more likely to develop diabetes; nevertheless, even in men, the pancreas may suffer significant damage from cancer or inflammation before its ability to produce insulin is compromised to the point that symptoms of an acute insulin shortage appear.

Because of the way the body is built, there is a safety factor for each organ. For example, illness can affect a very substantial portion of the liver before any functional impairment is apparent. The same is true for the heart and kidneys, and in the case of the pancreas, this safety factor explains why not everyone has diabetes. Very few people have a normal pancreas since inflammations of the organs close to it are rather prevalent (such as gallbladder inflammation), and these inflammations commonly involve the pancreas. Nonetheless, the proportion of people with diabetes who have documented gallbladder illness is not significantly higher than that of people who do not exhibit any signs of these inflammations.

Diabetes is brought on by arterial hardening. The pancreas, like all other organs in the body, can be harmed by disruptions in blood flow, particularly when the artery walls that supply it with blood become harder and its lumens, or channels, narrow. This is one way that diabetes can develop in older people with hardened arteries. Conversely, a large number of people without diabetes have severe vascular disease, which destroys the pancreatic islands as a result.

Diabetes can be caused by infections. Scarlet fever, mumps, influenza, or other common illnesses can contaminate the sensitive tissues of the pancreas, just as they might other organs. As a result, diabetes may arise from these illnesses. But there's nothing particular about this. It is true that some cases of diabetes can be linked to an acute intoxication of this type in the past, but diabetes is not invariably the result of any of the recognized viruses.

The main cause of diabetes is functional overstrain. Disease, particularly heart disease but also diseases of other organs, is known to be caused by functional overstrain. Overexertion can cause irreversible damage to the heart. A major cause of diabetes is functional overstrain of the pancreatic islands brought on by prolonged overindulgence. People who overeat often are typically noticeably overweight. For whatever reason that is still unknown, some individuals who are skinny can also be prone to overeating.

The norm is that overeating causes obesity, and it is a well-known fact that many diabetic patients are or have been overweight. Obesity is a sign of overeating and functional overstrain of the pancreas. For example, Dr. Joslin discovered that 75% of the 1,000 diabetic patients were either over or had been normal weight. It takes ten diabetic patients to make a ton of diabetes, according to Dr. Joslin. Among all the causes of diabetes, overeating with the accompanying long-term functional overstrain of Langerhans islets is most likely the most prevalent.

Sugar eating: It is significant that America's rising diabetes incidence and massive rise in sugar consumption are occurring at the same time. Between 1880 and 1890, each person used 44 pounds of sugar annually. It had increased to 84 pounds in 1921 and 103 pounds in 1922. Diabetes caused 5.5 deaths per 100,000 people in 1890; by 1921, that number had increased to 16.8 deaths per 100,000 people. Compared to practically all other foods, sugar is the easiest to overeat, and it's likely that sugar puts more functional strain on the pancreas than grains or fats do. Starches are easily absorbed into the bloodstream and cause the stomach to enlarge and full, which suppresses appetite. Sugar dissolves in water, moves swiftly through the stomach, absorbs nearly instantly, and immediately calls on the pancreas to work. Sweets are the usual desserts. Even when we are overindulged in meat and potatoes, there is always room for sweets, especially candies. The craze for soft drinks because the elimination of alcoholic beverages would undoubtedly lead to a rise in the number of new diabetes cases. I have seen a number of individuals whose extreme diabetes and coma were brought on abruptly by a soft drink binge.

Diabetes can strike without warning. Among younger people and kids, in particular, it often develops suddenly and seems to have no apparent trigger. As far as solid information indicates, these individuals' pancreas has never been inflamed; they are young and do not have vascular disease, and they have never been overweight or overindulged in food. How can we explain these children's and young people's diabetes? How can we explain why some obese people develop diabetes but not all do? How can we explain why some patients with very little pancreatic disease have diabetes while others have very extensive pancreatic destruction and do not?

Diabetes predisposition inherited from parents. The answer most likely lies somewhere in the murky world of heredity. Some of us have weak eyes from birth, while others have weak islands. The degree of inherent island weakness dictates the islands' vulnerability to functional overstrain from overindulging as well as to harm from infectious diseases or inadequate blood circulation. If a person has a significant predisposition to diabetes, diabetes may manifest in very early life. Here, the pancreas is not strong enough to endure the typical functional strain of growing. When this occurs, the illness is extremely severe. If a person has a small inclination for diabetes, it might not manifest itself unless they have a prolonged history of overeating. When the pancreatic islands operate well, they may resist infections, damage from illnesses, and inadequate blood flow; when they malfunction, diabetes arises. Although several family members with diabetes rarely develop the condition together, this does not imply that heredity cannot pass on the tendency. Many people who are seen as normal may possess this inclination without ever exhibiting any symptoms.

MEDICATION FOR DIABETES

Prevention: Nine diabetic people can be saved with a quick fix. Numerous diseases, including yellow fever, diphtheria, smallpox, and typhoid, have all but vanished. The white plague, often known as tuberculosis, is spreading quickly. Why not treat diabetes in the same way? Overeating has been shown to be the common cause. Thus, let us impart the benefits of maintaining a trim and healthy figure. By the way, this kind of instruction could aid in managing other long-term conditions. There's grounds to assume that obesity increases the risk of heart problems, high blood pressure, gallstones, and cancer compared to lean individuals.

Being obese is a sign of chronic overstrain on all body organs' functions. Particularly harmful to the pancreas is overindulging in proteins and carbs. The number of new diabetes patients in Berlin during the war significantly dropped, a time when the population's food supplies were severely restricted and sugar and meat in particular were in short supply. Diabetes is rapidly rising in America due to rising sugar consumption and rising levels of luxury. Not because they are Jewish, but rather because so many of them are luxury seekers, gluttons, and obese Jews, the Jewish people as a race have high rates of diabetes. Overeating cannot be completely avoided in order to eradicate diabetes. As we've shown, those who are thin may not be immune to a strong hereditary propensity; they may experience the most severe form of diabetes at a young age, but over time, even the frequency of these cases may decline. A reputable source once released the family trees of several families with diabetes, and these family trees indicate that the likelihood of developing diabetes increases with each generation. The grandparents' condition was minor and developed later in life, not until they were obese and had likely overindulged for a long time. Presumably due to less overeating, the condition was more severe and manifested earlier in life in the parents. In the third generation, children with even less provocation from overeating developed the condition. Therefore, by maintaining our fitness, perhaps we can prevent childhood diabetes, which is always severe and, thus, the most dreaded, and preserve our grandkids. A try is worthwhile.

Early case detection: Everybody should have a urine test on their birthday each year, according to Dr. Joslin, who has done more than anyone else to educate Americans with diabetes on staying well and strong. Thankfully, life insurance exams are now far more common than they were in the past, and they often identify many early cases of diabetes. After receiving the appropriate care, diabetic patients are instructed to do a urine sugar test. Every one of these has a responsibility to regularly check on the other family members. Why not give our high school chemistry students an easy test to complete and advise them to watch out for their family members?

Without a doubt, every druggist should be aware of the test and be prepared to provide it upon request for a little price.

Whether a patient sees a doctor early or late has a significant impact. With improved treatment techniques, early instances are being stabilized, if not completely cured. A few of these might be curable. It's still too early to tell. For patients who have had the condition for a long time, there is minimal chance of achieving curative outcomes or of strengthening a severely compromised pancreas.

Treatment: Based on specific concepts that make sense given the nature of the condition, the patient's care is provided.

Treatment guiding principles: If diabetes is caused, as appears most likely, by an overworked pancreas rendered weak by heredity, then reducing this strain is the apparent method to manage the condition. The exact same idea directs our treatment of cardiac disease. The benefits of physical rest are profound for the heart. For the pancreas, cautious dieting has the same effect. By structuring the diet in a way that minimizes the overall sugar content, or the burden on the pancreas, we are able to achieve three main goals: the elimination of sugar from the urine, a reduction of sugar in the blood, and the management of bothersome symptoms like frequent urination, excessive thirst, and skin dryness and itching. At the same time, we allow the pancreas to recuperate and become stronger.

Dietary measures can yield completely satisfactory outcomes in moderate cases of diabetes; the milder the illness, the less food restriction is required. Dietary therapy alone is less effective in severe cases of diabetes since it must be lowered to the point where the patient is malnourished. All such cases, prior to the discovery of insulin, presented a terrible dilemma. Either the patient could be fed, or the diet had to be restricted to the point where the patient actually starved to death; in the latter instance, death from diabetic coma was to be expected. Insulin is very helpful in these kinds of situations. With the use of insulin, severe cases of diabetes can be treated as moderate cases. Giving the patient enough extra insulin each day to increase his sugar tolerance is all that is needed. After that, he can resume his regular activities and enjoy normal strength and health with a cautious but sufficient diet. Diabetes is not being cured by this, but the worst of its fears are being banished.

It is impossible to ignore the diet. Some people might wonder why dieting is required when taking insulin. If it's true that the sole metabolic disruption associated with diabetes is insufficient insulin, then we should be able to fully remedy this error by providing enough insulin and allowing ourselves to eat anything we desire. Though theoretically valid, this is not practical for the reasons listed below.

About 300 grams, or 10 ounces, of carbohydrates, 150 grams, or 5 ounces, of protein, and 90 grams, or 3 ounces, of fat make up an unrestricted typical diet. Approximately 400 grams of sugar are produced during digestion, and 150 to 300 units of insulin are required to metabolize this quantity of sugar. An average person's pancreas likely produces 200–300 units of insulin each day, which is enough for any typical need. However, this naturally occurring insulin is delivered to the body's tissues gradually, ensuring that the blood never contains too much of it.

Excessive insulin is dangerous. In those with severe diabetes, the pancreas produces only 20 to 30 units of insulin each day, thus the remaining amount needs to be administered by hypodermic syringe in two or three doses. Each hypodermic injection would require 50 units of extra insulin if the daily total needed was 150 units, and it is challenging to administer such high doses without temporarily raising the blood insulin level. Regretfully, too much insulin is just as unpleasant as not enough insulin. An excessive amount of insulin causes the blood sugar to drop dangerously low, which can lead to a reaction with worrisome symptoms and potentially fatal outcomes. As a result, extremely excessive insulin doses should be avoided, and the daily intake of sugar should be tracked and adjusted to balance with insulin dosages. Dieting is required here.

Furthermore, when diets are extremely high in carbohydrates, it becomes exceedingly difficult to maintain low blood sugar levels using insulin. As I mentioned earlier, the typical sugar level is 0.1%. It can be as much as 0.5% or more in cases of uncontrolled diabetes. An insulin injection can lower this, but as soon as food high in carbohydrates is consumed, the sugar levels return to their elevated state. Blood sugar levels must be maintained low to allow the pancreas to rest, and this can only be done with a diet low in carbohydrates.

THE MENU

Low sugar and calorie intake is recommended. It is well acknowledged by the leading experts on diabetes that a patient with diabetes should not overeat and gain weight. Put otherwise, there needs to be a restriction on the overall energy, or calories, that come from food. It is also well acknowledged that a low-sugar diet is necessary. This indicates a low protein and carbohydrate content. As I've already mentioned, the health diet contains a lot of carbohydrates—possibly more than is prudent even for absolutely normal people. A diabetic diet needs to contain more fat in its calories and fewer grains and meats. Furthermore, authorities concur that severely limiting carbohydrates (sugar and starch) may be harmful since extremely low carb diets may cause lipids to not be adequately absorbed, which could lead to acid toxicity.

The authorities concur on broad guidelines. The exact diet-planning techniques used by different authorities vary only little and in specifics. For example, Dr. Allen is one of those who advocates for considerably stricter limits on the total amount of food consumed. Additionally, Dr. Joslin advocates for relatively low overall food intake and doesn't think that much fat should be allowed until very high amounts of carbohydrates can be consumed. Doctors McCann at the University of Rochester, New York, Dr. Woodyat of Chicago, and the physicians at the Toronto Clinic design their diets so that one part carbohydrates is consumed for every two and a half parts fat. Restricting protein is crucial, according to Professor Petren of Lund, Sweden, who is currently the foremost authority in Europe, as well as Doctors Newburgh and Marsh of the University of Michigan. If this is done, acidosis can be prevented even while feeding higher fat proportions. The Mayo Clinic practices strict dietary restrictions on protein and carbohydrates, which results in a diet that is primarily high in fat. However, this is planned so that the daily food supply's total energy content closely matches the patient's actual energy needs. The methods used to arrive at these many diets are documented in a number of patient handbooks.

Patient education books on diabetes include Lea and Febiger's "Diabetic Manual," written by Dr. Joslin. Another is "Diabetes, Its Treatment by Insulin and Diet," by Dr. Petty, published by the F. A. Davis Company in Philadelphia. For more thorough explanations of the techniques used in the Mayo Clinic than can be provided here, go to Wilder, Foley, and Ellithorpe's "A Primer for Diabetic Patients," published by W. B. Saunders Company in Philadelphia.

Patients need to be educated. Proper care produces results that are nearly as excellent as cures. They are not remedies because the underlying island weakness is seldom, if ever, fully fixed and requires month-long treatment. Therefore, the patient plays a major role in his or her own success, and the doctors' primary responsibility is to educate the patient on proper food and insulin use. The books listed were authored to aid with this patient education. Patients receive dietetics instruction and attend classes in various clinics around the nation until they are able to precisely weigh food and organize meals so that each one contains a specific number of calories and provides a specified amount of sugar for the metabolism. Until the patient is able to lead a healthy life despite having diabetes, the hospital's management of their condition is not over. Even if he may be brought back from the brink of death with insulin when he is in a coma at the hospital, he will relapse into the same risky situation when he returns home unless he has learnt how to continue taking the medication and mix it with a healthy diet.

It is always preferable to begin therapy in a hospital where a methodical education program can be acquired. Hospitals are the only educational options available to diabetes patients, which is unfortunate because some people detest hospitals. If one is lucky enough to see a doctor who will take the time to provide this instruction, they can achieve good outcomes at home. What are the prerequisites?

First and foremost, the patient needs to be able to read food tables and use them as a tool to construct precise diets. Food tables are listings of foods with their respective protein, carbohydrate, and fat compositions displayed. These lists are found in all of the works discussed here. The United States Department of Agriculture's Bulletin No. 28, "The Chemical Composition of American Food Materials," is the most comprehensive table available. It can be obtained for a nominal fee of ten cents from the Superintendent of Documents, Government Printing Office, Washington, D.C.

The second is instruction on how to use the hypodermic syringe and inject insulin. As previously mentioned, insulin must be administered hypodermically, or beneath the skin. The technique is simple, but sterile measures need to be taken to prevent contaminating the insulin with pathogens.

Third, guidance on performing a urine sugar test. This is a straightforward yet crucial task. Urine sugar is the first indicator of insufficient therapy. It would be foolish to wait to fix the error until further symptoms like thirst, frequent urination, and weakness manifest. The sugar test takes three minutes to conduct and should be performed daily, ideally using a urine sample that the patient passes right before going to bed. There should be no sugar on this specimen. If not, either the diet needs to be readjusted or additional insulin is required.

Fourth, suggestions on how to handle specific complexities that I will address later.

MANAGEMENT OF LOW-RISK DIABETES

Patients with diabetes have been known to survive for twenty years or longer without receiving any kind of medical care. The patient who suffers from a moderately severe or severe type of the disease should not be unwary despite this comforting concept. Overestimating the severity of the ailment is a safer course of action than making a mistake that cannot be undone and failing to take proper care of a critical condition. For example, children and young people may appear well in the first year following the emergence of sugar, but unless they receive very thorough treatment from the beginning, they almost always develop the severest form of the disease later.

Many elderly individuals can receive satisfactory treatment with far less food restriction than what is required in extreme instances. If this is achievable, there is no need for insulin and it should not be used; put another way, if a disease is severe enough to call for insulin, it is also severe enough to call for a diet that is precisely weighed. Sometimes patients are so illiterate that it is impossible to expect them to continue the weighed diet at home. In this case, as well as for individuals with extremely mild diabetes, the general recommendations listed below are typically helpful:

Steer clear of sugar and anything that has been sweetened with it, including candies, jam, marmalade, syrup, molasses, pies, cakes, puddings, and pastries. If desired, one-fourth grain saccharin has the same sweetening effect as one teaspoonful of sugar.

Steer clear of cereals for breakfast and cereal-based goods such noodles, mush, macaroni, and spaghetti.

Don't use more than one ounce of bread during a meal; instead, use it sparingly. Any bread that is marketed as "diabetes bread" is not as good as whole wheat or white bread. Because brown, corn, and gluten breads have such different compositions, it is safer to stay away from them.

Use little amounts of potatoes, bananas, apples, peas, dry beans, carrots, beets, turnips, and onions as often as once a day.

Avoiding dried fruits is advised. When feasible, use fresh fruit. Sugar-free fruit cans are acceptable. They can be made at home or bought from the market. You can replace other treats with fruits every day.

Eat enough of the vegetables that grow above ground, except peas and dry beans, to prevent hunger. You can have three regular servings of these veggies with every meal. Vegetables from cans are tasty and nutritious. On the other hand, fresh vegetables are better.

Eggs and meat ought to be consumed in moderation. Excess protein can cause just as much harm as excess carbohydrates. Never include more than 60 grams (2 ounces) of cooked, weighed lean meat and three eggs in your daily diet. You may add thirty grams (1 ounce) of cooked bacon, weighed after cooking. Fish, game, and chicken are examples of meat.

You can freely consume fats such as butter, oleomargarine, nut butter, bacon fat, olive oil, Wesson oil, or other salad oils.

For diabetics, cream is a highly helpful meal that may be consumed in moderation. Milk is less nutritious and has a comparatively high carbohydrate content.

To ensure that the amount of fat—such as butter or cream—provides sufficient but not excessive nourishment, it should be regulated. Less food is required when one's body weight is increasing, and in such cases, one should consume less fat.

Use of tea and coffee should be limited to no more than one cup each meal.

When used in moderation, condiments like vinegar, salt, and pepper are OK.

Bread should be avoided if there is evidence of sugar in the urine. If it still exists after cutting back on the amount of carbohydrates consumed, the patient's condition is serious enough to justify implementing the more precise management that is covered in this article.

THE MANAGEMENT OF FEVERS IN PATIENTS WITH DIABETES

Insulin is required more when a patient has a fever. With insulin, a patient on a good diet can now function and live like a normal neighbor. His inability to always subdue his enemy is a handicap, but if this control is vigilantly upheld, he ought to enjoy a life that is just as long and productive as that of his companions. But, he and his friends encounter illnesses other than diabetes throughout their lives. He will be attacked by measles, mumps, scarlet fever, diphtheria, acute colds, influenza, pneumonia, and other germ diseases, which are known as infectious diseases. When these illnesses strike, they always make his diabetes worse and put him at risk of acid poisoning from smoldering fats because they prevent his sugars from being used. Consequently, whether or not the patient had previously been able to go without insulin when such difficulties arise, they require it, and the doses required to manage these serious emergencies must typically be high. For example, a patient on a fixed diet who needs 20 units of insulin daily to keep his urine sugar-free may need to take 40 units every time he gets a cold. You might need to take 80 units of insulin each day if you have a serious infection like pneumonia. In most cases, a patient receiving 20 or 30 units of insulin per day responds extremely well to injections of 15 units each, given twice a day, one before breakfast and the other before dinner. Four injections spaced six hours apart may be required during a pneumonia episode or any other fever-producing problem. When a patient is ill, it is typically required to adjust and decrease the diet. Eating less is always a good idea. Specifically, the diet's fat limit ought to be lowered. Reducing the amount of carbohydrates is a bad idea. During the course of a fever, the patient may experience nausea and refuse all meals. In such cases, larger dosages of insulin are typically still required, but less may be needed. It's unclear why, but it seems that the toxins produced by bacterial infections negate the effects of insulin. Every six hours, the urine should be checked for illness, and the amount of sugar detected can be used to determine the appropriate insulin dosage.

DIABETIC PATIENT OPERATIONS

Particular care must be used while operating on diabetic patients.—It goes without saying that a person with diabetes has the same increased risk of appendicitis, gallstones, and cancer as a person without the disease. As a result, major surgeries are occasionally required. Unless their diabetes is carefully managed, diabetic people are far more at risk from these treatments than non-diabetic patients. In the past, one in three procedures on patients with diabetes ended in death. This was due to the fact that the anesthetic, either ether or chloroform, caused acid poisoning, and the weak patient was ill-prepared to handle the shock of blood loss and injury. The additional risk of diabetes can be prevented if the patient is well before the procedure and if acidosis is quickly treated with insulin. It is prudent for the patient with diabetes to only work with a highly skilled surgeon, and to ensure that he is either experienced in treating diabetes or has a physician with extensive experience treating diabetes associated with him.

Differential complications

Arteriosclerosis: As we get above the age of 38, we are able to enjoy a life that our grandparents were not able to. In 1860, a newborn baby's life expectancy was thirty-eight years. It has been almost sixty years now. This explains, in large part, why there has been a particularly sharp rise in the prevalence of diabetes among adults over 45 and why other chronic diseases are increasingly common nowadays. One of the most common complications among older diabetic patients is arteriosclerosis, or hardening of the arteries. As mentioned previously, in a predisposed individual, arteriosclerosis may be the cause of diabetes; nevertheless, diabetes itself aggravates and accelerates artery disease if left unchecked after it becomes established. Therefore, it is crucial that the elderly diabetic patient take his condition seriously and work to prevent arteriosclerosis by having his diabetes monitored. The majority of issues that plague and jeopardize elderly patients are brought on by artery hardening. In this illness, scar tissue gradually replaces the elastic contracting tissue in the hollow muscle tubes that convey blood.

What happens when the walls of the tubes thicken and crack? Apoplexy, cardiac problems, gangrene. Apoplexy can result from a cerebral hemorrhage or a cerebral artery break. In the eye, a vessel may potentially burst. The heart cannot receive enough blood through the constricted tubes to keep pounding, which causes angina, irregular heartbeat, or even heart failure. This restricts circulation in the legs, causing pain and occasionally even gangrene. It will be remembered that among younger diabetic patients, coma is the leading cause of death. Nowadays, coma is preventable, and no one should pass away from coma. The leading cause of death for elderly patients is gangrene. The tissues of gangrene, which typically affects the legs, become lifeless due to a shortage of blood; infection ensues, ultimately leading to blood poisoning.

Prevent gangrene: We need to stop these gangrene-related deaths. Vigilance and focus can help achieve this. The first requirement is to keep the urine sugar-free. It is possible to induce healing in gangrenous ulcers of the feet by rigorous insulin therapy and diet. Encouraging the circulation in the feet with massage and appropriate exercises is very important. Ultimately, taking precautions to shield the skin on your feet from cuts and bruises will save a lot of trouble. Every elderly diabetes patient should wear highly comfortable shoes, clean stockings, and wash his feet every day. Keep an eye on and protect the feet. The Greek warrior Achilles had to have had diabetes. His heel was the lone weak point in his body. He died when Paris' spear touched his heel in front of Troy's fortifications. Keep an eye on and protect the feet.